Ketogenic Air Fryer Essential Recipes

A Collection of Delicious Ketogenic Air Fryer Recipes for Your Daily Meals

Morgan Parry

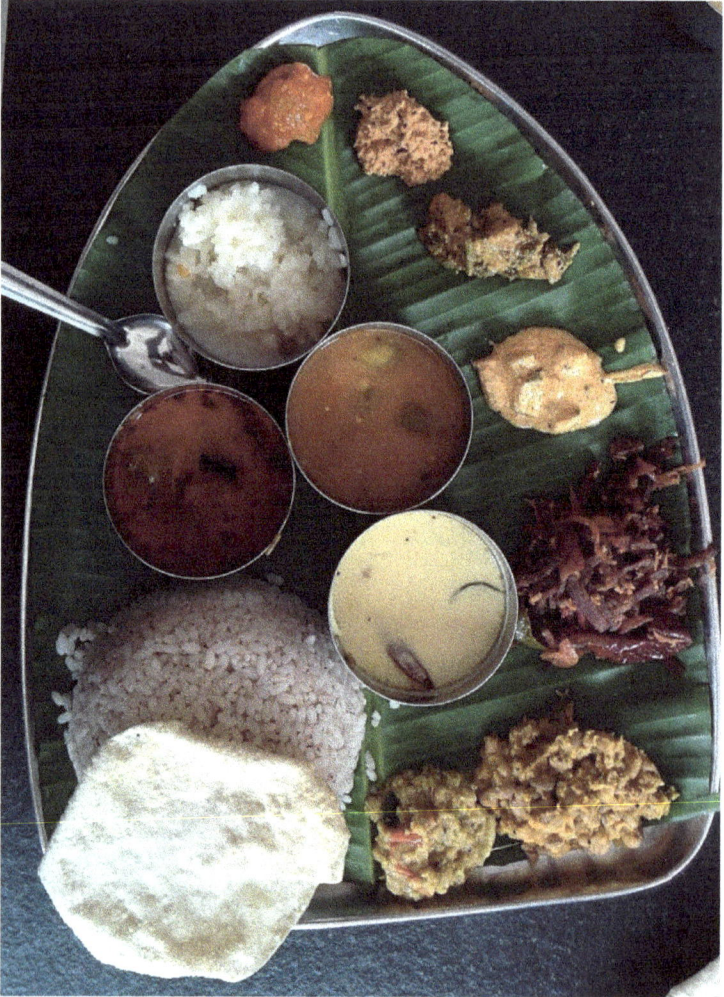

advice. The content within this book has been derived from various sources. Please consult a licensed professional before attempting any techniques outlined in this book.

By reading this document, the reader agrees that under no circumstances is the author responsible for any losses, direct or indirect, which are incurred as a result of the use of information contained within this document, including, but not limited to, — errors, omissions, or inaccuracies.

Table of Contents

Beef Pie

Prep time: 25 minutes

Cooking time: 6 minutes

Servings: 4

Ingredients:

- 2 cup cauliflower, boiled, mashed

- 2 oz celery stalk, chopped

- 1 cup ground beef

- ½ teaspoon salt

- ½ teaspoon ground turmeric

- 1 tablespoon coconut oil

- ½ teaspoon avocado oil

- 1 teaspoon dried parsley

- 1 tablespoon keto tomato sauce

- 1 garlic clove, diced

Directions:

1.   Toss the coconut oil in the skillet and melt it over the medium heat. Then add celery stalk. Cook the vegetables for 5 minutes. Stir them from time to time. Meanwhile, brush the air fryer pan with avocado oil. Transfer the cooked vegetables in the pan and flatten them in the shape of the layer.

2.   Then put the ground beef in the pan. Add salt, parsley, and turmeric. Cook the ground meat for 10 minutes over the medium heat. Stir it from time to time. Add tomato sauce and stir well. After this, transfer the ground beef over the vegetables. Then add garlic and top the pie with mashed cauliflower mash. Preheat the air fryer to 360F. Put the pan with shepherd pie in the air fryer and cook for 6 minutes or until you get the crunchy crust.

Nutrition: calories 116, fat 7.7, fiber 1.9, carbs 4.5, protein 7.8

Paprika Chicken

Preparation time: 10 minutes

Cooking time: 35 minutes

Servings: 6

Ingredients:

• 3 pounds chicken thighs, bone-in

• ½ cup butter, melted

• 1 tablespoon smoked paprika 1 teaspoon lemon juice

Directions:

1. In a bowl, mix the chicken thighs with the paprika, toss, put all the pieces in your air fryer's basket and cook them at 360 degrees F for 25 minutes shaking the fryer from time to time and basting the meat with the butter. Divide between plates and serve.

Nutrition: calories 261, fat 16, fiber 3, carbs 5, protein 12

Creamy Zucchini Noodle Mix

Prep time: 10 minutes

Cooking time: 9 minutes

Servings: 2

Ingredients:

- 1 zucchini, trimmed

- 4 oz chicken breast, skinless, boneless

- ¼ cup heavy cream

- 2 oz Parmesan, grated

- ½ teaspoon ground black pepper

- ¼ teaspoon ground paprika

- ½ teaspoon sesame oil

- ½ teaspoon dried basil

Directions:

1. Make the zoodles from the zucchini with the help of the spiralizer. Then rub the chicken breast with ground black pepper, paprika, and basil.

2.   Sprinkle the chicken breast with sesame oil and put it in the air fryer. Cook it for 8 minutes at 400F. Flip the chicken on another side after 4 minutes of cooking. When the chicken is cooked, remove it from the air fryer and place it on the plate. Then put the zucchini zoodles in the air fryer and cook then at 400F for 1 minute. Meanwhile, mix up parmesan and heavy cream and preheat the liquid over the medium heat until the cheese is melted. Then mix up heavy cream sauce and zucchini. Mix it up well. Chop the chicken roughly and top the zoodles with it.

Nutrition: calories 235, fat 14.4, fiber 1.3, carbs 5.2, protein 22.7

Tomato Cod Bake

Preparation time: 5 minutes

Cooking time: 12 minutes

Servings: 4

Ingredients:

- tablespoons butter, melted

- 2 tablespoons parsley, chopped

- ¼ cup keto tomato sauce 8 cherry tomatoes, halved

- 2 cod fillets, boneless, skinless and cubed Salt and black pepper to the taste

Directions:

1. In a baking pan that fits the air fryer, combine all the Ingredients, toss, put the pan in the machine and cook the mix at 390 degrees F for 12 minutes. Divide the mix into bowls and serve for lunch.

Nutrition: calories 232, fat 8, fiber 2, carbs 5, protein 11

Wrapped Zucchini

Prep time: 10 minutes

Cooking time: 10 minutes

Servings: 2

Ingredients:

- 2 zucchinis, trimmed
- 8 bacon slices
- 1 teaspoon sesame oil
- ¼ teaspoon chili powder

Directions:

1.   Cut every zucchini into 4 sticks and sprinkle with chili powder. Then wrap every zucchini stick in bacon and sprinkle with sesame oil. Preheat the air fryer to 400F. Put the zucchini sticks in the air fryer in one layer and cook for 10 minutes. Flip the zucchini sticks after 5 minutes of cooking.

Nutrition: calories 464, fat 34.4, fiber 2.3, carbs 7.8, protein 30.6

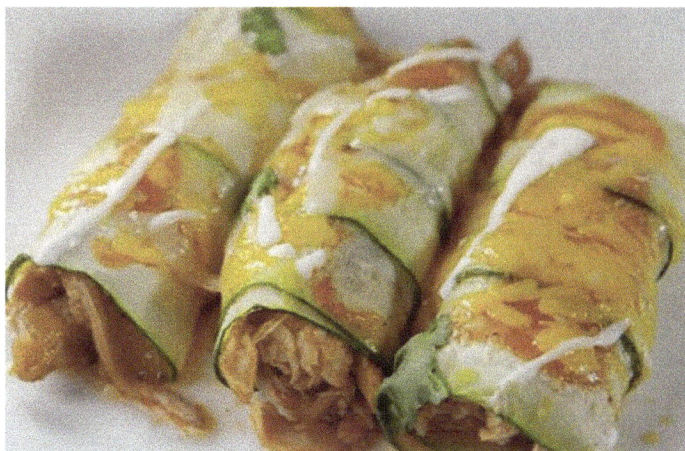

Parsley Turkey Stew

Preparation time: 5 minutes

Cooking time: 25 minutes

Servings: 4

Ingredients:

•   1 turkey breast, skinless, boneless and cubed 1 tablespoon olive oil

•   1 broccoli head, florets separated 1 cup keto tomato sauce

•   Salt and black pepper to the taste 1 tablespoon parsley, chopped

Directions:

1.   In a baking dish that fits your air fryer, mix the turkey with the rest of the Ingredients except the parsley, toss, introduce the dish in the fryer, bake at 380 degrees F for 25 minutes, divide into bowls, sprinkle the parsley on top and serve.

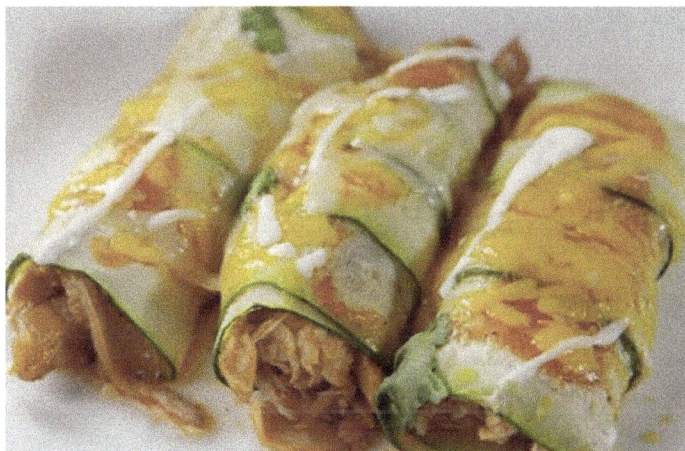

Parsley Turkey Stew

Preparation time: 5 minutes

Cooking time: 25 minutes

Servings: 4

Ingredients:

- 1 turkey breast, skinless, boneless and cubed 1 tablespoon olive oil

- 1 broccoli head, florets separated 1 cup keto tomato sauce

- Salt and black pepper to the taste 1 tablespoon parsley, chopped

Directions:

1. In a baking dish that fits your air fryer, mix the turkey with the rest of the Ingredients except the parsley, toss, introduce the dish in the fryer, bake at 380 degrees F for 25 minutes, divide into bowls, sprinkle the parsley on top and serve.

Nutrition: calories 250, fat 11, fiber 2, carbs 6, protein 12

Creamy Zucchini Noodle Mix

Prep time: 10 minutes

Cooking time: 9 minutes

Servings: 2

Ingredients:

- 1 zucchini, trimmed

- 4 oz chicken breast, skinless, boneless

- ¼ cup heavy cream

- 2 oz Parmesan, grated

- ½ teaspoon ground black pepper

- ¼ teaspoon ground paprika

- ½ teaspoon sesame oil

- ½ teaspoon dried basil

Directions:

3.   Make the zoodles from the zucchini with the help of the spiralizer. Then rub the chicken breast with ground black pepper, paprika, and basil.

4.   Sprinkle the chicken breast with sesame oil and put it in the air fryer. Cook it for 8 minutes at 400F. Flip the chicken on another side after 4 minutes of cooking. When the chicken is cooked, remove it from the air fryer and place it on the plate. Then put the zucchini zoodles in the air fryer and cook then at 400F for 1 minute. Meanwhile, mix up parmesan and heavy cream and preheat the liquid over the medium heat until the cheese is melted. Then mix up heavy cream sauce and zucchini. Mix it up well. Chop the chicken roughly and top the zoodles with it.

Nutrition: calories 235, fat 14.4, fiber 1.3, carbs 5.2, protein 22.7

Crab Stuffed Flounder

Prep time: 10 minutes

Cooking time: 12 minutes

Servings: 3

Ingredients:

- 9 oz flounder fillets
- 4 oz crab meat, chopped
- 1 tablespoon mascarpone
- ½ teaspoon ground nutmeg
- 2 spring onions, diced
- ½ teaspoon dried thyme
- 2 oz Parmesan, grated
- 1 egg, beaten

Directions:

1.   Line the air fryer baking pan with baking paper. After this, cut the flounder fillet on3 servings and transfer them in the baking pan in one layer. Sprinkle the fish

fillets with ground nutmeg and dried thyme. Then top them with chopped crab meat, spring onions, and Parmesan. In the mixing bowl, mix up mascarpone and egg. Pour the liquid over the cheese. Preheat the air fryer to 385F. Place the baking pan with fish in the air fryer and cook the meal for 12 minutes.

Nutrition: calories 230, fat 8.3, fiber 0.3, carbs 2.8, protein 33.9

Butter Paprika Swordfish

Preparation time: 5 minutes

Cooking time: 12 minutes

Servings: 4

Ingredients:

- 4 swordfish fillets, boneless 1 tablespoon olive oil

- ¾ teaspoon sweet paprika 2 teaspoons basil, dried Juice of 1 lemon

- 2 tablespoons butter, melted

Directions:

1. In a bowl, mix the oil with the other Ingredients except the fish fillets and whisk. Brush the fish with this mix, place it in your air fryer's basket and cook for 6 minutes on each side. Divide between plates and serve with a side salad.

Nutrition: calories 216, fat 11, fiber 3, carbs 6, protein 12

Caribbean Ginger Sea bass

Prep time: 15 minutes

Cooking time: 10 minutes

Servings: 2

Ingredients:

- ¼ habanero, chopped

- 1 teaspoon Caribbean spices

- 8 oz sea bass, trimmed

- ½ teaspoon Erythritol

- 1 teaspoon smoked paprika

- ¼ teaspoon minced ginger

- 1 tablespoon avocado oil

Directions:

1.   In the mixing bowl mix up Caribbean spices, Erythritol, and smoked paprika. Then rub the sea bass with the spice mixture well. In the shallow bowl, whisk together minced ginger and avocado oil. Brush the fish

with the ginger mixture. Preheat the air fryer to 400F. Put the sea bass in the air fryer and cook it for 10 minutes.

Nutrition: calories 291, fat 8.3, fiber 1.1, carbs 9.4, protein 0.4

Trout and Shallots

Preparation time: 5 minutes

Cooking time: 12 minutes

Servings: 4

Ingredients:

- 4 trout fillets, boneless Juice of 1 lime
- ½ cup butter, melted
- ½ cup olive oil
- garlic cloves, minced 6 shallots, chopped
- A pinch of salt and black pepper

Directions:

1. In a pan that fits the air fryer, combine the fish with the shallots and the rest of the Ingredients, toss gently, put the pan in the machine and cook at 390 degrees F for 12 minutes, flipping the fish halfway. Divide between plates and serve with a side salad.

Nutrition: calories 270, fat 12, fiber 4, carbs 6, protein 12

Lemon Branzino

Prep time: 10 minutes

Cooking time: 8 minutes

Servings: 4

Ingredients:

- 1-pound branzino, trimmed, washed
- 1 teaspoon Cajun seasoning
- 1 tablespoon sesame oil
- 1 tablespoon lemon juice
- 1 teaspoon salt

Directions:

1.   Rub the branzino with salt and Cajun seasoning carefully. Then sprinkle the fish with the lemon juice and sesame oil. Preheat the air fryer to 380F. Place the fish in the air fryer and cook it for 8 minutes.

Nutrition: calories 141, fat 5.9, fiber 0, carbs 0.1, protein 21

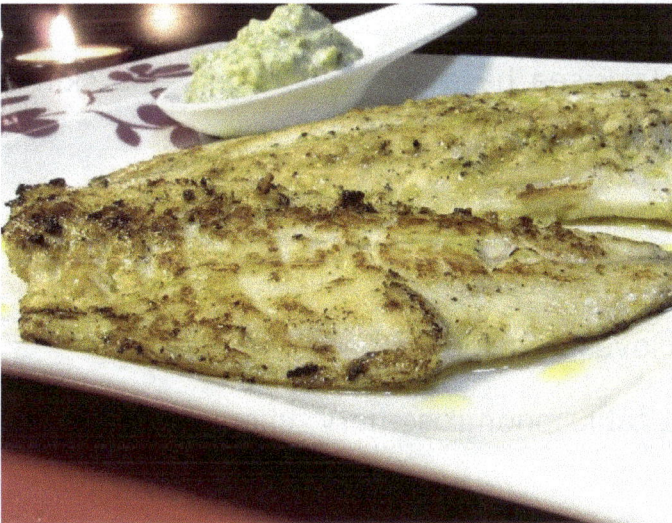

Sea Bass with Vinaigrette

Preparation time: 5 minutes

Cooking time: 12 minutes

Servings: 4

Ingredients:

• black sea bass fillets, boneless and skin scored 2 tablespoons olive oil

• A pinch of salt and black pepper

• 3 tablespoons black olives, pitted and chopped 3 garlic cloves, minced

• 1 tablespoon rosemary, chopped Juice of 1 lime

Directions:

1. In a bowl, mix the oil with the olives and the rest of the Ingredients except the fish and whisk well. Place the fish in a pan that fits the air fryer, spread the rosemary vinaigrette all over, put the pan in the machine and cook at 380 degrees F for 12 minutes, flipping the fish halfway. Divide between plates and serve.

Nutrition: calories 220, fat 12, fiber 4, carbs 6, protein 10

Chili Squid Rings

Prep time: 15 minutes

Cooking time: 10 minutes

Servings: 2

Ingredients:

- 8 oz squid tube, trimmed, washed

- 4 oz chorizo, chopped

- 1 teaspoon olive oil

- 1 teaspoon chili flakes

- 1 tablespoon keto mayonnaise

Directions:

1. Preheat the air fryer to 400F and put the chopped chorizo in the air fryer basket. Sprinkle it with chili flakes and olive oil and cook for 6 minutes. Then shake chorizo well. Slice the squid tube into the rings and add in the air fryer. Cook the meal for 4 minutes at 400F. Shake the cooked meal well and transfer it in the plates. Sprinkle the meal with keto mayonnaise.

Nutrition: calories 338, fat 25.5, fiber 0, carbs 1.1, protein 25.7

Trout and Tomato Zucchinis Mix

Preparation time: 5 minutes

Cooking time: 15 minutes

Servings: 4

Ingredients:

- 3 zucchinis, cut in medium chunks 4 trout fillets, boneless
- 2 tablespoons olive oil
- ¼ cup keto tomato sauce
- Salt and black pepper to the taste 1 garlic clove, minced
- tablespoon lemon juice
- ½ cup cilantro, chopped

Directions:

1. In a pan that fits your air fryer, mix the fish with the other Ingredients, toss, introduce in the fryer and cook at 380 degrees F for 15 minutes. Divide everything between plates and serve right away.

Nutrition: calories 220, fat 12, fiber 4, carbs 6, protein 9

Chicken and Rice Casserole

Preparation time: 5 minutes

Cooking time: 35 minutes

Servings: 4

Ingredients:

- cups cauliflower florets, chopped A pinch of salt and black pepper

- A drizzle of olive oil

- 6 ounces coconut cream

- 2 tablespoons butter, melted 2 teaspoons thyme, chopped 1 garlic clove, minced

- 1 tablespoon parsley, chopped

- 4 chicken thighs, boneless and skinless

Directions:

1. Heat up a pan with the butter over medium heat, add the cream and the other Ingredients except the cauliflower, oil and the chicken, whisk, bring to a simmer and cook for 5 minutes. Heat up a pan with the oil over

medium-high heat, add the chicken and brown for 2 minutes on each side. In a baking dish that fits the air fryer, mix the chicken with the cauliflower, spread the coconut cream mix all over, put the pan in the machine and cook at 380 degrees F for 20 minutes. Divide between plates and serve hot.

Nutrition: calories 280, fat 14, fiber 4, carbs 6, protein 20

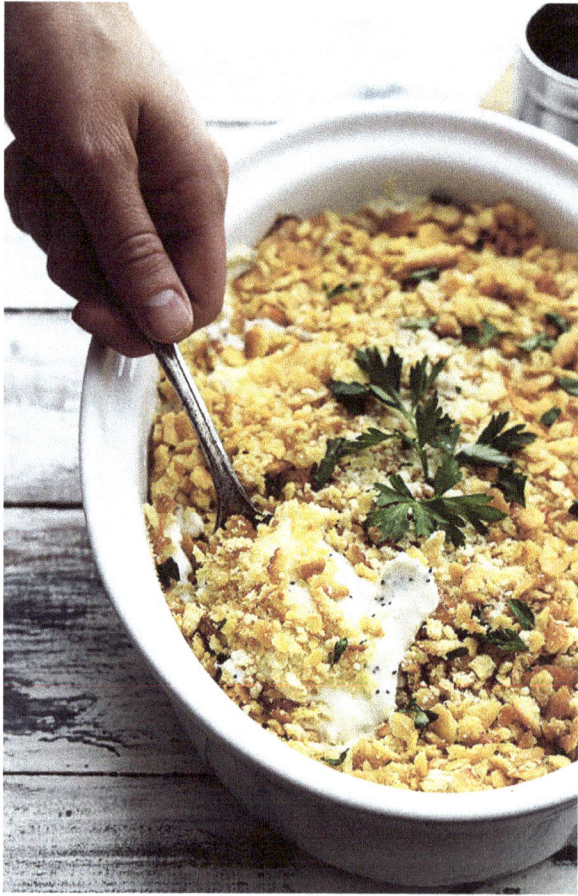

Hazelnut Crusted Chicken

Prep time: 10 minutes

Cooking time: 10 minutes

Servings: 4

Ingredients:

- 1-pound chicken fillet
- 3 oz hazelnuts, grinded
- 2 egg whites, whisked
- ½ teaspoon ground black pepper
- ½ teaspoon salt
- 1 tablespoon coconut flour
- 1 teaspoon avocado oil

Directions:

1. Cut the chicken on 4 tenders and sprinkle them with ground black pepper and salt. In the mixing bowl mix up grinded hazelnuts and coconut flour. Then dip the chicken tenders in the whisked egg and coat in the

hazelnut mixture. Sprinkle every chicken tender with avocado oil. Preheat the air fryer to 365F. Place the prepared chicken tenders in the preheated air fryer and cook for 10 minutes.

Nutrition: calories 369, fat 21.8, fiber 2.9, carbs 5, protein 38.2

Oregano Chicken and Green Beans

Preparation time: 5 minutes

Cooking time: 35 minutes

Servings: 4

Ingredients:

- 4 chicken breasts, skinless, boneless and halved 10 ounces chicken stock

- 1 teaspoon oregano, dried

- 10 ounces green beans, trimmed and halved 2 tablespoons olive oil

- A pinch of salt and black pepper 1 tablespoon parsley, chopped

Directions:

1. Heat up a pan that fits the air fryer with the oil over medium-high heat, add the chicken and brown for 2 minutes on each side. Add the remaining Ingredients, toss a bit, put the pan in the machine and cook at 380

degrees F for 30 minutes. Divide everything between plates and serve.

Nutrition: calories 241, fat 11, fiber 5, carbs 6, protein 14

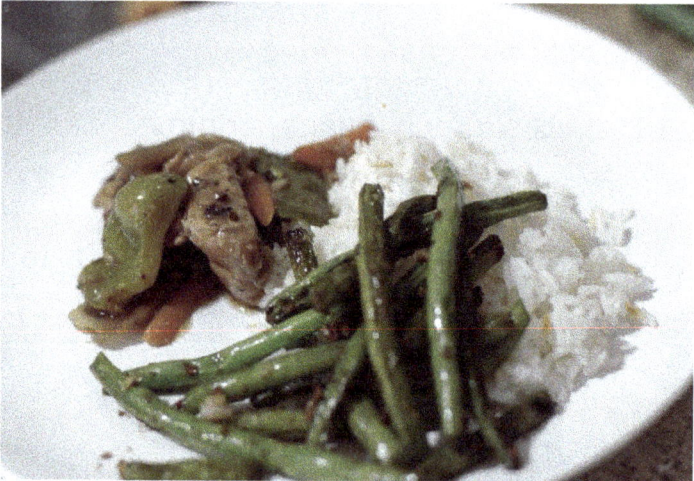

Pesto Chicken

Prep time: 10 minutes

Cooking time: 25 minutes

Servings: 4

Ingredients:

- 12 oz chicken legs
- 1 teaspoon sesame oil
- ½ teaspoon chili flakes
- 4 teaspoons pesto sauce

Directions:

1.   In the shallow bowl mix up pesto sauce, chili flakes, and sesame oil. Then rub the chicken legs with the pesto mixture. Preheat the air fryer to 390F. Put the chicken legs in the air fryer basket and cook them for 25 minutes.

Nutrition: calories 194, fat 9.6, fiber 0.1, carbs 0.3, protein 25.1

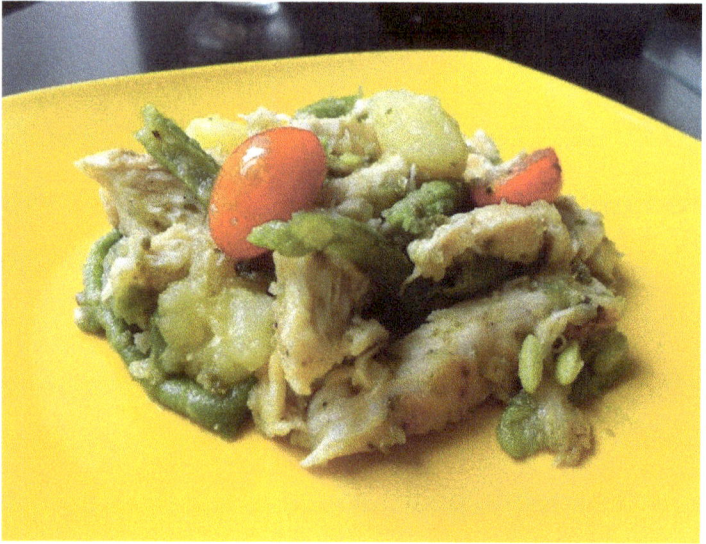

Chicken with Tomatoes and Peppers

Preparation time: 5 minutes

Cooking time: 25 minutes

Servings: 4

Ingredients:

- 4 chicken breasts, skinless, boneless and halved 2 zucchinis, sliced

- 4 tomatoes, cut into wedges

- 2 yellow bell peppers, cut into wedges 2 tablespoons olive oil

- 1 teaspoon Italian seasoning

Directions:

1. In a baking dish that fits your air fryer, mix all the Ingredients, toss, introduce in the fryer and cook at 380 degrees F for 25 minutes. Divide everything between plates and serve.

Nutrition: calories 280, fat 12, fiber 4, carbs 6, protein 14

Creamy Duck and Lemon Sauce

Preparation time: 5 minutes

Cooking time: 25 minutes

Servings: 4

Ingredients:

- 2 spring onions, chopped

- 2 tablespoons butter, melted 4 garlic cloves, minced

- 1 and ½ teaspoons coriander, ground Salt and black pepper to the taste

- 15 ounces tomatoes, crushed

- ¼ cup lemon juice

- and ½ pounds duck breast, skinless, boneless and cubed

- ½ cup cilantro, chopped

- ½ cup chicken stock

- ½ cup heavy cream

Directions:

1.　　Heat up a pan that fits your air fryer with the butter over medium heat, add the duck pieces and cook for 5 minutes. Add the rest of the ingredients except the cilantro, toss, introduce the pan in the fryer and cook at 370 degrees F for 20 minutes. Divide between plates and serve.

Nutrition: calorie 284, fat 12, fiber 4, carbs 6, protein 17

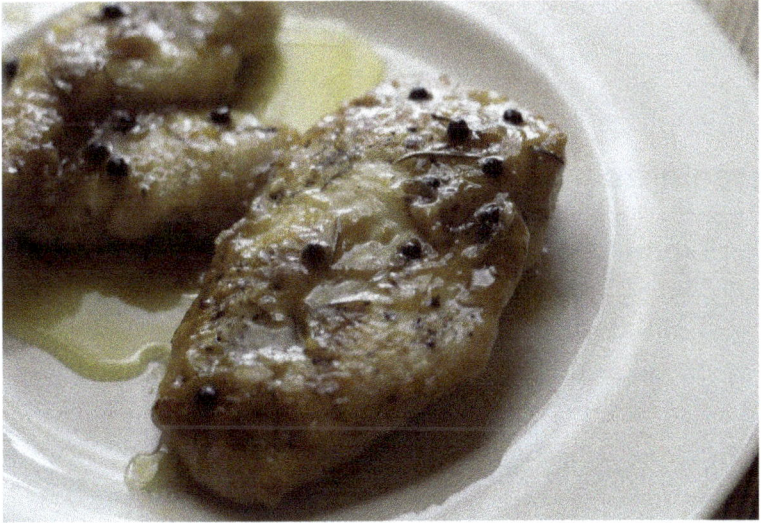

Paprika Liver Spread

Prep time: 10 minutes

Cooking time: 8 minutes

Servings: 6

Ingredients:

- 1-pound chicken liver

- 2 tablespoons ghee

- 1 teaspoon salt

- 1 teaspoon smoked paprika

- ¼ cup hot water

Directions:

1.   Preheat the air fryer to 400F. Wash and trim the chicken liver and arrange it in the air fryer basket. Cook the Ingredients for 5 minutes. Then flip them on another side and cook for 3 minutes more. When the chicken liver is cooked, transfer it in the blender. Add ghee, salt, and smoked paprika. Add hot water and blend the mixture

until smooth. Then transfer the cooked chicken pâté in the bowl and store it in the fridge for up to 3 days.

Nutrition: calories 167, fat 9.2, fiber 0.3, carbs 1.4, protein 18.6

Pork and Peppers Mix

Preparation time: 5 minutes

Cooking time: 25 minutes

Servings: 4

Ingredients:

- 1 pound pork tenderloin, sliced

- ¼ cup cilantro, chopped

- ½ teaspoon garlic powder 1 tablespoon olive oil

- 1 green bell pepper, julienned

- ½ teaspoon chili powder

- ½ teaspoon cumin, ground

Directions:

1.	Heat up a pan that fits the air fryer with the oil over medium heat, add the pork and brown for 5 minutes. Add the rest of the Ingredients, toss, put the pan in the air fryer and cook at 400 degrees F for 20 minutes. Divide between plates and serve.

Nutrition: calories 284, fat 13, fiber 4, carbs 6, protein 17

Cardamom Lamb Mix

Prep time: 30 minutes

Cooking time: 20 minutes

Servings: 2

Ingredients:

- 10 oz lamb sirloin

- 1 oz fresh ginger, sliced

- 2 oz spring onions, chopped

- ¼ teaspoon ground cinnamon

- ½ teaspoon ground cardamom

- ½ teaspoon fennel seeds

- ½ teaspoon chili flakes

- ¼ teaspoon salt

- 1 tablespoon avocado oil

Directions:

1.   Put the fresh ginger in the blender. Add onion, ground cardamom, cinnamon, fennel seeds, chili flakes,

salt, and avocado oil. Blend the mixture until you get the smooth mass. After this, make the small cuts in the lamb sirloin. Rub the meat with the blended spice mixture and leave it for 20 minutes to marinate. Meanwhile, preheat the air fryer to 350F. Put the marinated lamb sirloin in the air fryer and cook it for 20 minutes. Flip the meat on another side in halfway. Slice the cooked meat.

Nutrition: calories 355, fat 18.8, fiber 1.1, carbs 7, protein 36.6

Creamy Pork Mix

Preparation time: 5 minutes

Cooking time: 25 minutes

Servings: 4

Ingredients:

- 1 pound pork stew meat, cubed 4 teaspoons sweet paprika
- A pinch of salt and black pepper 1 cup coconut cream
- 1 tablespoon butter, melted
- 1 tablespoon parsley, chopped

Directions:

1. Heat up a pan that fits the air fryer with the butter over medium heat, add the meat and brown for 5 minutes. Add the remaining Ingredients, toss, put the pan in the air fryer, cook at 390 degrees F for 20 minutes more, divide into bowls and serve.

Nutrition: calories 273, fat 12, fiber 4, carbs 6, protein 20

Smoked Pork

Prep time: 20 minutes

Cooking time: 20 minutes

Servings: 5

Ingredients:

- 1-pound pork shoulder
- 1 tablespoon liquid smoke
- 1 tablespoon olive oil
- 1 teaspoon salt

Directions:

1.   Mix up liquid smoke, salt, and olive oil in the shallow bowl. Then carefully brush the pork shoulder with the liquid smoke mixture from each side. Make the small cuts in the meat. Preheat the air fryer to 390F. Put the pork shoulder in the air fryer basket and cook the meat for 10 minutes. After this, flip the meat on another side and cook it for 10 minutes more.

2.   Let the cooked pork shoulder rest for 10-15 minutes. Shred it with the help of 2 forks.

Nutrition: calories 289, fat 22.2, fiber 0, carbs 0, protein 21.1

Balsamic Pork Chops

Preparation time: 5 minutes

Cooking time: 25 minutes

Servings: 4

Ingredients:

- 4 pork chops
- tablespoon smoked paprika 1 tablespoon olive oil
- tablespoons balsamic vinegar
- ½ cup chicken stock
- A pinch of salt and black pepper

Directions:

1.   In a bowl, mix the pork chops with the rest of the Ingredients and toss. Put the pork chops in your air fryer's basket and cook at 390 degrees F for 25 minutes. Divide between plates and serve.

Nutrition: calories 276, fat 12, fiber 4, carbs 6, protein 22

Coconut Fried Mushrooms

Prep time: 10 minutes

Cooking time: 5 minutes

Servings: 2

Ingredients:

- 6 oz white mushrooms

- 2 tablespoons almond flour

- 1 teaspoon coconut flour

- ½ teaspoon sesame oil

- ½ teaspoon salt

- 1 tablespoon cream cheese

- ½ teaspoon ground nutmeg

Directions:

1.   Trim the mushrooms and sprinkle with salt and ground nutmeg. Then mix up mushrooms and cream cheese. In the bowl mix up almond flour and coconut flour. Coat the mushrooms in the coconut flour mixture.

Preheat the air fryer to 400F. Put the mushrooms in the air fryer and sprinkle with sesame oil. Cook the mushrooms for 5 minutes.

Nutrition: calories 214, fat 17.5, fiber 4.5, carbs 9.9, protein 9.3

Parsley Savoy Cabbage Mix

Preparation time: 5 minutes

Cooking time: 15 minutes

Servings: 4

Ingredients:

• Savoy cabbage, shredded 2 spring onions, chopped

• tablespoons keto tomato sauce Salt and black pepper to the taste 1 tablespoon parsley, chopped

Directions:

1. In a pan that fits your air fryer, mix the cabbage the rest of the ingredients except the parsley, toss, put the pan in the fryer and cook at 360 degrees F for 15 minutes. Divide between plates and serve with parsley sprinkled on top.

Nutrition: calories 163, fat 4, fiber 3, carbs 6, protein 7

Coconut Walnuts

Preparation time: 5 minutes

Cooking time: 40 minutes

Servings: 12

Ingredients:

- 1 and ¼ cups almond flour 1 cup swerve
- 1 cup butter, melted
- ½ cup coconut cream
- 1 and ½ cups coconut, flaked 1 egg yolk
- ¾ cup walnuts, chopped
- ½ teaspoon vanilla extract

Directions:

1. In a bowl, mix the flour with half of the swerve and half of the butter, stir well and press this on the bottom of a baking pan that fits the air fryer.

2. Introduce this in the air fryer and cook at 350 degrees F for 15 minutes. Meanwhile, heat up a pan with the rest of the butter over medium heat, add the remaining swerve and the rest of the Ingredients, whisk,

cook for 1-2 minutes, take off the heat and cool down. Spread this well over the crust, put the pan in the air fryer again and cook at 350 degrees F for 25 minutes. Cool down, cut into bars and serve.

Nutrition: calories 182, fat 12, fiber 2, carbs 4, protein 4

Buttery Muffins

Prep time: 15 minutes

Cooking time: 10 minutes

Servings: 2

Ingredients:

- 1 teaspoon of cocoa powder

- 2 tablespoons coconut flour

- 2 teaspoons swerve

- ½ teaspoon vanilla extract

- 2 teaspoons almond butter, melted

- ¼ teaspoon baking powder

- 1 teaspoon apple cider vinegar

- ¼ teaspoon ground cinnamon

Directions:

1.   In the mixing bowl mix up cocoa powder, coconut flour, swerve, vanilla extract, almond butter, baking

powder, and apple cider vinegar. Then add ground cinnamon and stir the mixture with the help of the spoon until it is smooth. Pour the brownie mixture in the muffin molds and leave for 10 minutes to rest. Meanwhile, preheat the air fryer to 365F. Put the muffins in the air fryer basket and cook them for 10 minutes. Then remove the cooked brownie muffins from the air fryer and cool them completely.

Nutrition: calories 145, fat 10.4, fiber 5, carbs 10.7, protein 5.1

Lemon Butter Bars

Preparation time: 10 minutes

Cooking time: 35 minutes

Servings: 8

Ingredients:

- ½ cup butter, melted 1 cup erythritol

- and ¾ cups almond flour 3 eggs, whisked

- Zest of 1 lemon, grated Juice of 3 lemons

Directions:

1.   In a bowl, mIx 1 cup flour with half of the erythritol and the butter, stir well and press into a baking dish that fits the air fryer lined with parchment paper. Put the dish in your air fryer and cook at 350 degrees F for 10 minutes. Meanwhile, in a bowl, mix the rest of the flour with the remaining erythritol and the other Ingredients and whisk well. Spread this over the crust, put the dish in the air fryer once more and cook at 350 degrees F for 25 minutes. Cool down, cut into bars and serve.

Nutrition: calories 210, fat 12, fiber 1, carbs 4, protein 8

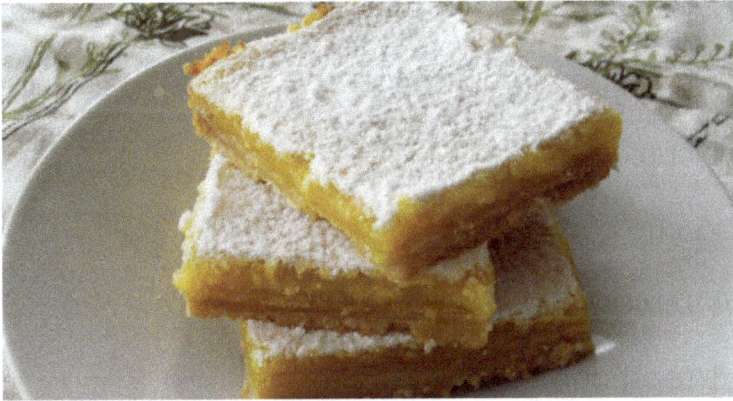

Nut Bars

Prep time: 15 minutes

Cooking time: 30 minutes

Servings: 10

Ingredients:

- ½ cup coconut oil, softened

- 1 teaspoon baking powder

- 1 teaspoon lemon juice

- 1 cup almond flour

- ½ cup coconut flour

- 3 tablespoons Erythritol

- 1 teaspoon vanilla extract

- 2 eggs, beaten

- 2 oz hazelnuts, chopped

- 1 oz macadamia nuts, chopped

- Cooking spray

Directions:

1.   In the mixing bowl mix up coconut oil and baking powder. Add lemon juice, almond flour, coconut flour, Erythritol, vanilla extract, and eggs. Stir the mixture until it is smooth or use the immersion blender for this step. Then add hazelnuts and macadamia nuts. Stir the mixture until homogenous. After this, preheat the air fryer to 325F. Line the air fryer basket with baking paper. Then pour the nut mixture in the air fryer basket and flatten it well with the help of the spatula. Cook the mixture for 30 minutes. Then cool the mixture well and cut it into the serving bars.

Nutrition: calories 208, fat 19.8, fiber 3.5, carbs 9.5, protein 4

Aromatic Cup

Prep time: 10 minutes

Cooking time: 15 minutes

Servings: 1

Ingredients:

- 1 egg, beaten
- 1 tablespoon peanut butter
- ½ teaspoon baking powder
- 1 teaspoon lemon juice
- ½ teaspoon vanilla extract
- 1 teaspoon Erythritol
- 2 tablespoons coconut flour

Directions:

1. Mix up all Ingredients in the cup until homogenous. Then preheat the air fryer to 350F. Put the cup with blondies in the air fryer and cook it for 15 minutes.

Nutrition: calories 237, fat 15, fiber 7, carbs 14, protein 12.6

Chocolate Ramekins

Preparation time: 5 minutes

Cooking time: 15 minutes

Servings: 6

Ingredients:

- cup blackberries

- eggs

- ½ cup heavy cream

- ½ cup ghee, melted

- ¼ cup chocolate, melted 1 tablespoons stevia

- 2 teaspoons baking powder

Directions:

1.   In a bowl, mix the blackberries with the rest of the ingredients, whisk well, divide into ramekins, put them in the fryer and cook at 340 degrees F for 15 minutes. Serve cold.

2.

Nutrition: calories 150, fat 2, fiber 2, carbs 4, protein 7

Cocoa Spread

Prep time: 10 minutes

Cooking time: 5 minutes

Servings: 4

Ingredients:

- 2 oz walnuts, chopped
- 5 teaspoons coconut oil
- ½ teaspoon vanilla extract
- 1 tablespoon Erythritol
- 1 teaspoon of cocoa powder

Directions:

1. Preheat the air fryer to 350F. Put the walnuts in the mason jar. Add coconut oil, vanilla extract, Erythritol, and cocoa powder. Stir the mixture until smooth with the help of the spoon. Then place the mason jar with Nutella in the preheated air fryer and cook it for 5 minutes. Stir Nutella before serving.

Ginger Vanilla Cookies

Preparation time: 10 minutes

Cooking time: 15 minutes

Servings: 12

Ingredients:

- 2 cups almond flour 1 cup swerve

- ¼ cup butter, melted 1 egg

- 2 teaspoons ginger, grated 1 teaspoon vanilla extract

- ¼ teaspoon nutmeg, ground

- ¼ teaspoon cinnamon powder

Directions:

1. In a bowl, mix all the Ingredients and whisk well. Spoon small balls out of this mix on a lined baking sheet that fits the air fryer lined with parchment paper and flatten them. Put the sheet in the fryer and cook at 360 degrees F for 15 minutes. Cool the cookies down and serve.

Nutrition: calories 220, fat 13, fiber 2, carbs 4, protein 3

Vanilla Mozzarella Balls

Prep time: 20 minutes

Cooking time: 4 minutes

Servings: 8

Ingredients:

- 2 eggs, beaten
- 1 teaspoon almond butter, melted
- 7 oz coconut flour
- 2 oz almond flour
- 5 oz Mozzarella, shredded
- 1 tablespoon butter
- 2 tablespoons swerve
- 1 teaspoon baking powder
- ½ teaspoon vanilla extract
- Cooking spray

Directions:

1.   In the mixing bowl mix up butter and Mozzarella. Microwave the mixture for 10-15 minutes or until it is melted. Then add almond flour and coconut flour. Add swerve and baking powder. After this, add vanilla extract and stir the mixture. Knead the soft dough. Microwave the mixture for 2-5 seconds more if it is not melted enough. In the bowl mix up almond butter and eggs. Make 8 balls from the almond flour mixture and coat them in the egg mixture. Preheat the air fryer to 400F. Spray the air fryer basket with cooking spray from inside and place the bread rolls in one layer.

2.   Cook the dessert for 4 minutes or until the bread roll is golden brown. Cool the cooked dessert completely and sprinkle with Splenda if desired.

Nutrition: calories 249, fat 14.4, fiber 10.9, carbs 8.3, protein 13.3

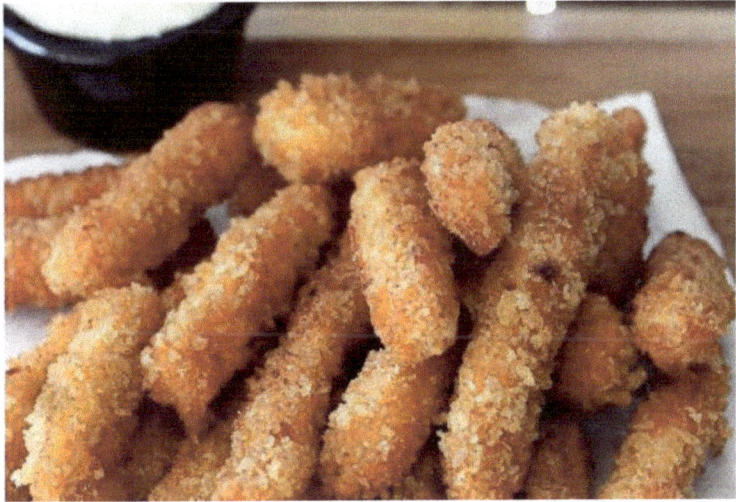

Cinnamon Raspberry Cupcakes

Preparation time: 10 minutes

Cooking time: 20 minutes

Servings: 8

Ingredients:

- ¾ cup raspberries
- ¼ cup ghee, melted 1 egg
- ½ cup swerve
- ¼ cup coconut flour
- 2 tablespoons almond meal
- 1 teaspoon cinnamon powder 3 tablespoons cream cheese
- ½ teaspoon baking soda
- ½ teaspoon baking powder Cooking spray

Directions:

1.   In a bowl, mix all the Ingredients except the cooking spray and whisk well. Grease a cupcake pan that

fits the air fryer with the cooking spray, pour the raspberry mix, put the pan in the machine and cook at 350 degrees F for 20 minutes. Serve the cupcakes cold.

Nutrition: calories 223, fat 7, fiber 2, carbs 4, protein 5

Raspberry Pop-Tarts

Prep time: 25 minutes

Cooking time: 10 minutes

Servings: 5

Ingredients:

- 2 oz raspberries

- ½ cup almond flour

- 1 egg, beaten

- 1 tablespoon butter, softened

- 1 tablespoon Erythritol

- ½ teaspoon baking powder

- 1 egg white, whisked

- Cooking spray

Directions:

1.   In the mixing bowl mix up almond flour, egg, butter, and baking powder Knead the soft non-sticky dough. Then mash the raspberries and mix them up with

Erythritol. Cut the dough into halves. Then roll up every dough half into the big squares. After this, cut every square into 5 small squares. Put the mashed raspberry mixture on 5 mini squares. Then cover them with remaining dough squares. Secure the edges with the help of the fork. Then brush the pop-tarts with whisked egg white. Preheat the air fryer to 350F. Spray the air fryer basket with cooking spray, then place the pop tarts in the air fryer basket in one layer. Cook them at 350F for 10 minutes. Cool the cooked pop-tarts totally and transfer in the serving plates.

Nutrition: calories 59, fat 4.7, fiber 1.1, carbs 2.3, protein 2.6

Lemon Berry Jam

Preparation time: 10 minutes

Cooking time: 20 minutes

Servings: 12

Ingredients:

- ¼ cup swerve

- 8 ounces strawberries, sliced 1 tablespoon lemon juice

- ¼ cup water

Directions:

1. In a pan that fits the air fryer, combine all the Ingredients, put the pan in the machine and cook at 380 degrees F for 20 minutes. Divide the mix into cups, cool down and serve.

Nutrition: calories 100, fat 1, fiber 0, carbs 1, protein 1

Creamy Raspberry Cake

Prep time: 20 minutes

Cooking time: 30 minutes

Servings: 4

Ingredients:

- 3 eggs, beaten

- ½ cup coconut flour

- ½ teaspoon baking powder

- 2 teaspoons Erythritol

- 1 teaspoon vanilla extract

- 1 tablespoon Truvia

- ½ cup heavy cream

- 1 oz raspberries, sliced

- Cooking spray

Directions:

1.   Make the cake batter: in the mixing bowl mix up beaten egg, coconut flour, baking powder, and Erythritol.

Add vanilla extract and stir the mixture until smooth. Then preheat the air fryer to 330F. Spray the air fryer baking pan with cooking spray and pour the cake batter inside. Put the pan with batter in the preheated air fryer and cook it for 30 minutes. Meanwhile, make the cake frosting: whip the heavy cream. Then add Truvia and stir it well. When the cake is cooked, cool it well and remove it from the air fryer pan. Slice the cake into 2 cakes. Then spread one piece of cake with ½ part of whipped cream and top with sliced raspberries.

2.   After this, cover it with the second piece of cakes. Top the cake with the remaining whipped cream.

Nutrition: calories 166, fat 10.9, fiber 5.5, carbs 11.1, protein 6.6

Blackberry Cream

Preparation time: 4 minutes

Cooking time: 20 minutes

Servings: 6

Ingredients:

- 2 cups blackberries Juice of ½ lemon
- 2 tablespoons water
- teaspoon vanilla extract 2 tablespoons swerve

Directions:

1. In a bowl, mix all the Ingredients and whisk well. Divide this into 6 ramekins, put them in the air fryer and cook at 340 degrees F for 20 minutes Cool down and serve.

Nutrition: calories 123, fat 2, fiber 2, carbs 4, protein 3

Coconut Almond Pies

Prep time: 25 minutes

Cooking time: 26 minutes

Servings: 6

Ingredients:

- 8 oz almond flour

- 1 teaspoon vanilla extract

- ¼ teaspoon salt

- 2 tablespoons Erythritol

- 2 eggs, beaten

- 1 tablespoon coconut butter, melted

- 1 tablespoon xanthan gum

- 1 teaspoon flax meal

- 2 oz blueberries

- Cooking spray

Directions:

1.	In the mixing bowl mix up vanilla extract, eggs, and coconut butter. Then add almond flour, salt, xanthan gum, and flax meal. Knead the non-sticky dough and roll it up. Then cut the dough on 6 pieces. Put the blueberries on every dough piece. Sprinkle the berries with Erythritol. Fold the dough pieces to make the pockets and secure the edges of them with the help of the fork. Preheat the air fryer to 350F. Place the hand pies in the air fryer in one layer (4 pies) and cook them for 13 minutes. Then remove the cooked pies from the air fryer and cool them to the room temperature.

2.	Repeat the same steps with remaining uncooked pies.

Nutrition: calories 270, fat 21.8, fiber 7.7, carbs 13, protein 10

Coconut Tomato

Preparation time: 3 minutes

Cooking time: 5 minutes

Servings: 4

Ingredients:

• 1/3 cup coconut cream

• ½ pound cherry tomatoes, halved

• avocados, pitted, peeled and cubed A pinch of salt and black pepper Cooking spray

Directions:

1. Grease the air fryer with cooking spray, combine the tomatoes with avocados, and the other Ingredients and cook at 350 degrees F for 5 minutes shaking once. Divide into bowls and serve.

Nutrition: calories 226, fat 12, fiber 2, carbs 4, protein 8

Eggplant Lasagna

Prep time: 20 minutes

Cooking time: 30 minutes

Servings: 6

Ingredients:

- 2 medium eggplants
- ½ cup keto tomato sauce
- 1 cup Cheddar cheese, shredded
- ½ cup Mozzarella cheese, shredded
- 1 cup ground pork
- 1 teaspoon Italian seasonings
- 1 teaspoon sesame oil

Directions:

1.   Slice the eggplants into the long slices. Then brush the air fryer pan with sesame oil. In the mixing bowl mix up ground pork and Italian seasonings. Then make the layer from the sliced eggplants in the air fryer pan. Top

it with a small amount of ground pork and mozzarella cheese. Then sprinkle mozzarella with the tomato sauce Place the second eggplant layer over the sauce and repeat all the steps again. Cover the last layer with remaining eggplant and top with Cheddar cheese. Cover the lasagna with foil and place it in the air fryer. Cook the meal for 20 minutes at 365F. Then remove the foil from the lasagna and cook it for 10 minutes more. Let the cooked lasagna cool for 10 minutes before serving.

Nutrition: calories 260, fat 18.7, fiber 0.8, carbs 3, protein 19.6

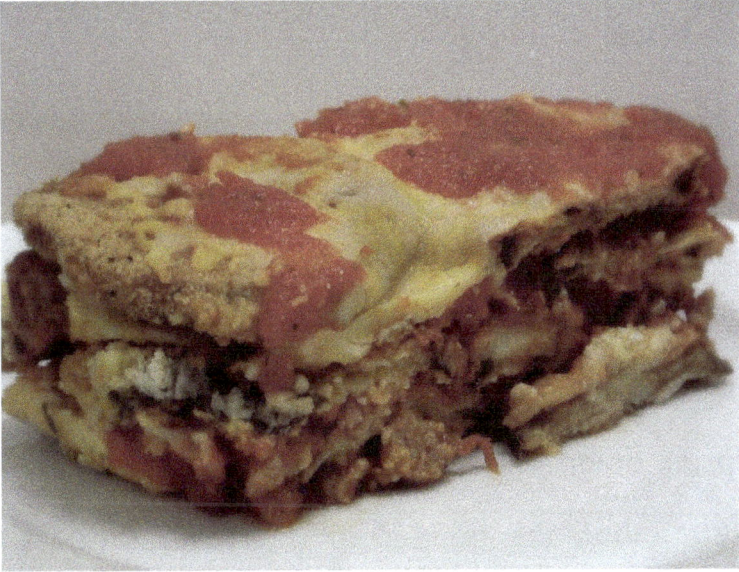

Pork and Mushrooms Mix

Preparation time: 5 minutes

Cooking time: 20 minutes

Servings: 4

Ingredients:

- pound pork stew meat, ground 1 cup mushrooms, sliced

- spring onions, chopped

- Salt and black pepper to the taste 1 teaspoon Italian seasoning

- ½ teaspoon garlic powder 1 tablespoon olive oil

Directions:

1.   Heat up a pan that fits the air fryer with the oil over medium high heat, add the meat and brown for 3-4 minutes. Add the rest of the Ingredients, stir, put the pan in the Air Fryer, cover and cook at 360 degrees F for 15 minutes. Divide between plates and serve for lunch.

Nutrition: calories 220, fat 12, fiber 2, carbs 4, protein 7

Italian Sausages

Prep time: 10 minutes

Cooking time: 12 minutes

Servings: 4

Ingredients:

- 4 pork Italian sausages
- ½ cup keto tomato sauce
- 4 Mozzarella sticks
- 1 teaspoon butter, softened

Directions:

1. Make the cross-section in every sausage with the help of the knife. Then fill the cut with the Mozzarella stick. Brush the air fryer pan with butter. Put the stuffed sausages in the pan and sprinkle them with tomato sauce. Preheat the air fryer to 375F. Place the pan with sausages in the air fryer and cook them for 12 minutes or until the sausages are golden brown.

Nutrition: calories 383, fat 29, fiber 0.3, carbs 5.8, protein 23.9

Parmesan Chicken

Preparation time: 5 minutes

Cooking time: 30 minutes

Servings: 4

Ingredients:

- 1 teaspoon olive oil

- 4 spring onions, chopped

- 2 chicken breasts, skinless, boneless and cubed
Salt and black pepper to the taste

- and ½ cups parmesan cheese, grated

- ½ cup keto tomato sauce

Directions:

1.   Preheat your air fryer at 400 degrees F, add half of the oil and the spring onions and fry them for 8 minutes, shaking the fryer halfway. Add the rest of the Ingredients, toss, cook at 370 degrees F for 22 minutes, shaking the fryer halfway as well. Divide between plates and serve for lunch.

Nutrition: calories 270, fat 14, fiber 2, carbs 6, protein 12

Chicken and Arugula Salad

Prep time: 15 minutes

Cooking time: 12 minutes

Servings: 2

Ingredients:

- 2 bacon slices, cooked, chopped

- 2 cups arugula, chopped

- 10 oz chicken breast, skinless, boneless

- 1 teaspoon ground black pepper

- ½ teaspoon salt

- 1 teaspoon avocado oil

- ½ teaspoon ground cumin

- ½ teaspoon ground paprika

- 1 tablespoon olive oil

- ¼ teaspoon minced garlic

- 1 teaspoon fresh cilantro, chopped

Directions:

1.   Rub the chicken breast with ground black pepper, salt, ground cumin, ground paprika, and avocado oil. Then preheat the air fryer to 365F. Put the chicken breast in the preheated air fryer and cook for 12 minutes.

2.   Meanwhile, in the salad bowl mix up chopped bacon, arugula, and fresh cilantro. In the shallow bowl mix up minced garlic and olive oil. Chop the cooked chicken breasts and add in the salad mixture. Sprinkle the salad with garlic oil and shake well.

Nutrition: calories 339, fat 19.1, fiber 1, carbs 2.5, protein 37.9

Pork and Eggs Bowls

Preparation time: 10 minutes

Cooking time: 15 minutes

Servings: 4

Ingredients:

- eggs, whisked

- 1 and ½ pounds pork meat, ground 2 teaspoons olive oil

- ½ cup keto tomato sauce

- Salt and black pepper to the taste

Directions:

1.   Heat up a pan that fits the Air Fryer with the oil over medium-high heat, add the meat and brown for 3-4 minutes. Add the rest of the ingredients, toss, put the pan in the machine and cook at 370 degrees F for 12 minutes. Divide into bowls and serve for lunch with a side salad.

2.

Nutrition: calories 270, fat 13, fiber 2, carbs 6, protein 8

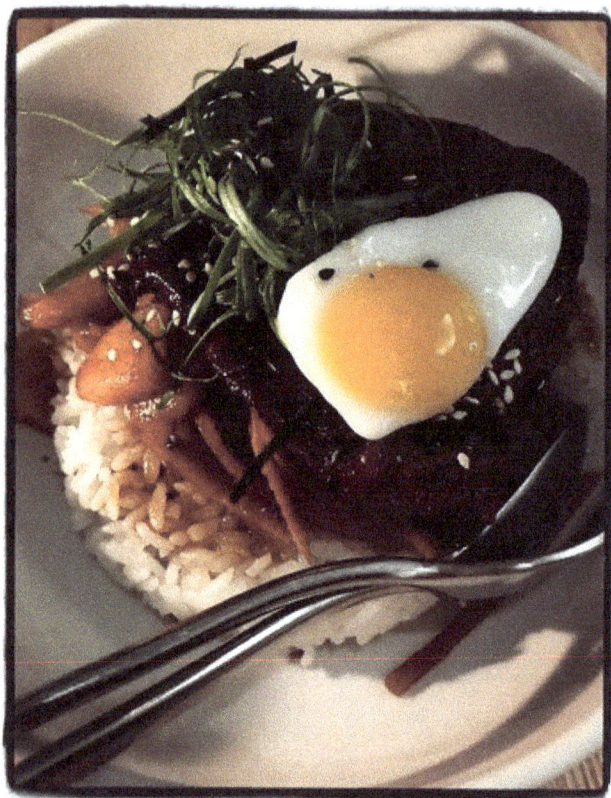

www.ingramcontent.com/pod-product-compliance
Lightning Source LLC
Chambersburg PA
CBHW050751030426
42336CB00012B/1765